TARA COLLINS

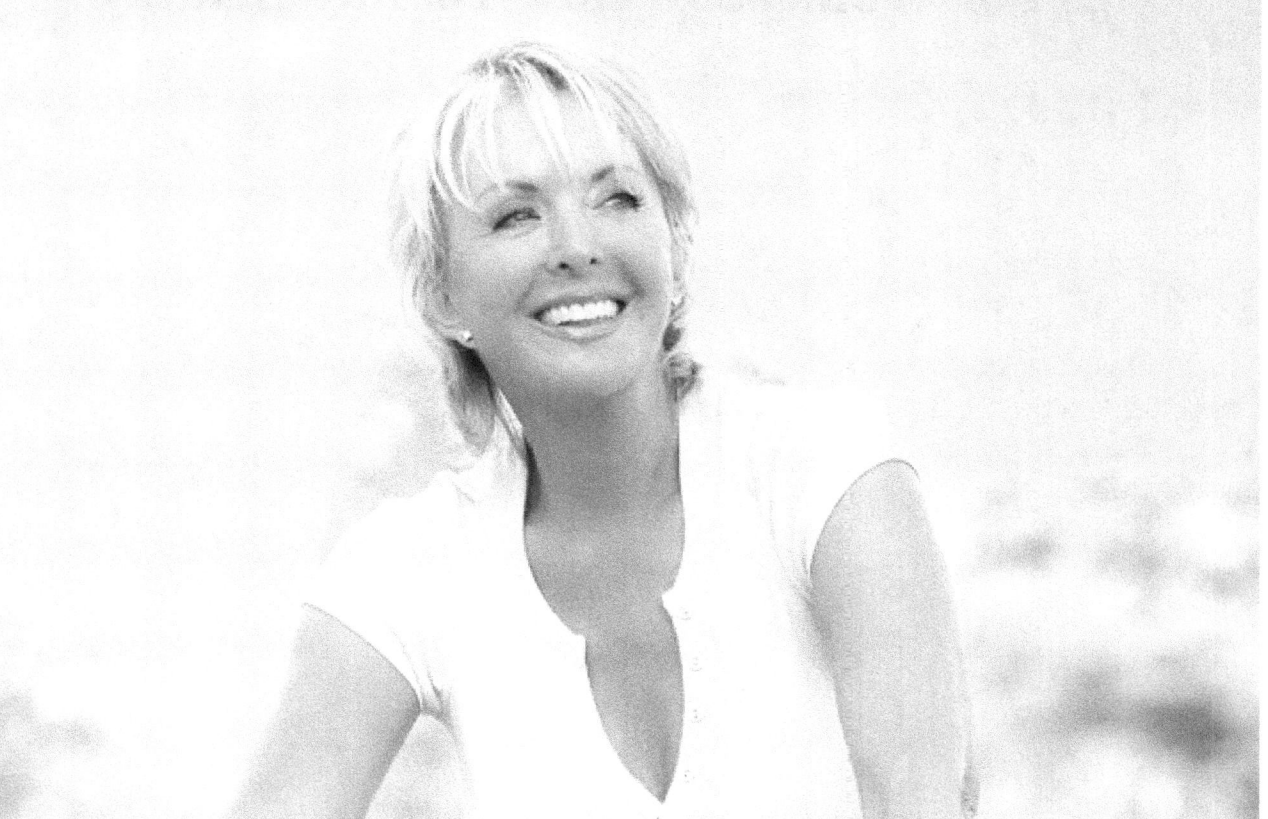

tips for *Women* on how to stay healthy

Tips For Women On How To Stay Healthy

By

Tara Collins

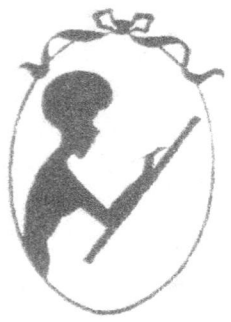

Published by Dane Print publication

Connect with me on FaceBook

https://www.facebook.com/pages/How-To-Stay-Healthy/294340720675061?ref=hl

The advice given in this book is only that of the author who has read and studied a lot about women's health. You should always consider medical advice for any ailments or serious problem you may have.

Table Of Content

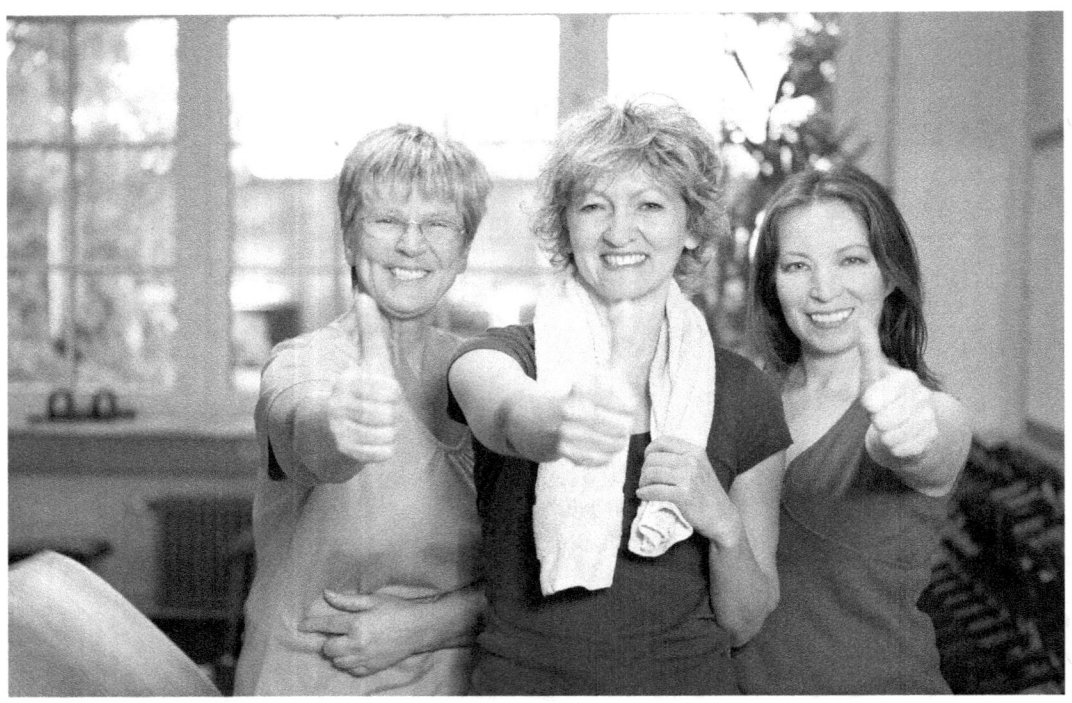

Introduction

Woman's body is a wonderful creation and all women should be proud to be a woman when we think of how creative we are. We can grow a baby and breast feed it in the early stages of the baby's life. A woman's body is like a temple and if you treat it with care on a regular basis in the correct way, many illnesses can be avoided. Sometimes we do need medical professionals to help us, but they are only part of the process to get you back to health. In the end you are the only one responsible for your health and well-being.

If you are going to be healthy then it is up to you to take the steps toward it. There is nothing magical that any book, motivational speaker, or video can tell you that is going to spark your interest into successfully improving your health. The only way that you can make your health better and keep yourself healthy on a permanent basis – is for you to decide that now is the time to do it.

Women come in all shapes and sizes and if we are not happy with the way we look there are lots of things we can do to improve our looks if we want it badly enough. However it is so important that you love yourself for who you are regardless of your looks, because the way you feel inside about yourself will shine through on the outer. You will have a glow of self acceptance shining through in your face and the energy you send out.

What do we mean by being healthy?

The question you may like to ask is what is being healthy really like? Does it mean that we have to be a super woman who does exercises and works out every day or runs marathon races? Or does it mean that you have to do meditation every day at a certain time so you can feel good inside? It will mean a different thing to every woman and whatever way you want to describe healthy is what it personally means to you.

Do You Listen To Your Body?

In this day and age most women are so busy that they have no time to listen to their bodies. Oh yes, they get aches and pains but they are too busy to pay attention to the signals their bodies are sending them. These are warning signs and it is the way your body is trying to make you aware of something in your body that needs a bit of tender loving care from you.

Your body may be run down and therefore your immune system is not functioning like it normally would and you may get ill more often than you used to. Illness very rarely come out of nowhere although you might think so, but the warnings have been there for a while, you just haven't paid attention to the signs your body has been giving you. However, if you listen to your body you may realize that your body is sending signals to you of an impending illness.

Your body, mind and spirit is not something individual or separate from each other, they are all part of you and you need to listen to whatever they are telling you. Most of us get a little ache or pain here and there and we don't have to run to the doctor every time that happens. But learn to listen to your body and get a feel of what it is telling you. Are you eating the right foods that agree with your body, do you need to get more fit, do you need medical care? If you learn to tune into your body then you will save yourself from many a heart ache.

****

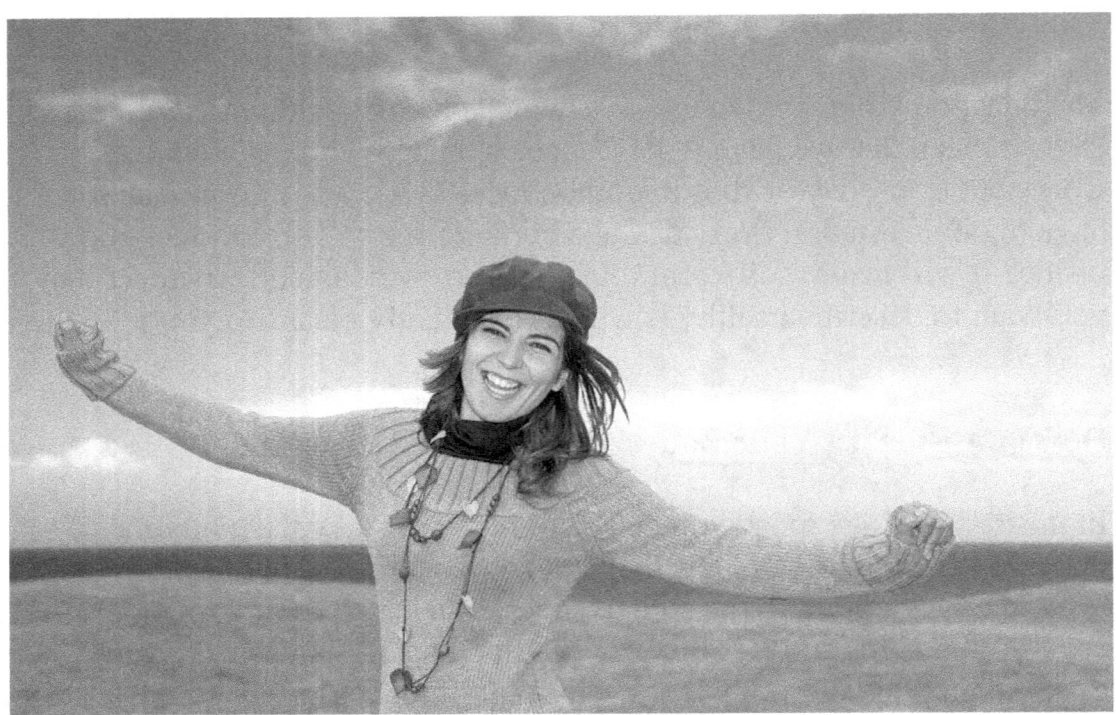

Keep your spirit up

If you are one of those unfortunate persons who suffer from a chronic condition that you have no control over, then you should do your best to keep your spirit up and never give up hope of getting better. Many people have been diagnosed with a condition that would never heal, but through hard work and an optimistic outlook they manage to get well and improve their health.

Don't let your mind tell you that it is impossible because then your body will start to believe the messages you are sending it. It is good to surround yourself with positive people but in the end, it is you who has to believe that you will get better and be strong.

Some women always seem to be healthy and hardly ever get sick. This can of course have a lot to do with their genes, but it also has to do with their outlook on life. They usually have an optimistic outlook on life and can always see the positive in everything and therefore their spirit is always up. Even though you are one of these fortunate women who are always healthy, it should be remembered that you do need to go to the doctor for a routine check up once in a while just to make sure everything is fine.

Keep a harmonious balance

For the best health for your body, you have to keep as harmonious a balance as possible in all areas of your life. Whether you have a family to look after or if you are a career woman, there will be times when life seems to become more stressful than normal and even the healthiest of women can come down with a cold. The thing to realize is that your brain will influence your body and if your stress level gets too high, it will be crucial to your health and a simple cold can be hard to get rid of. We loose touch with what our inner guidance system is telling us and we are not in touch with the things we ought to say no to.

To release some of your stress you should take 10 to 20 minutes during the day to relax yourself and do a simple meditation so you again can find a harmonious balance in your everyday life. It will help you to be more in touch with your inner feelings. So when someone asks for your help or wants you to do something and you are not quite sure how you feel about it, you should stop for a moment and check with your body and see if there is any part of it that tenses up; do you get a gut feeling of whether to say No or Yes?

****

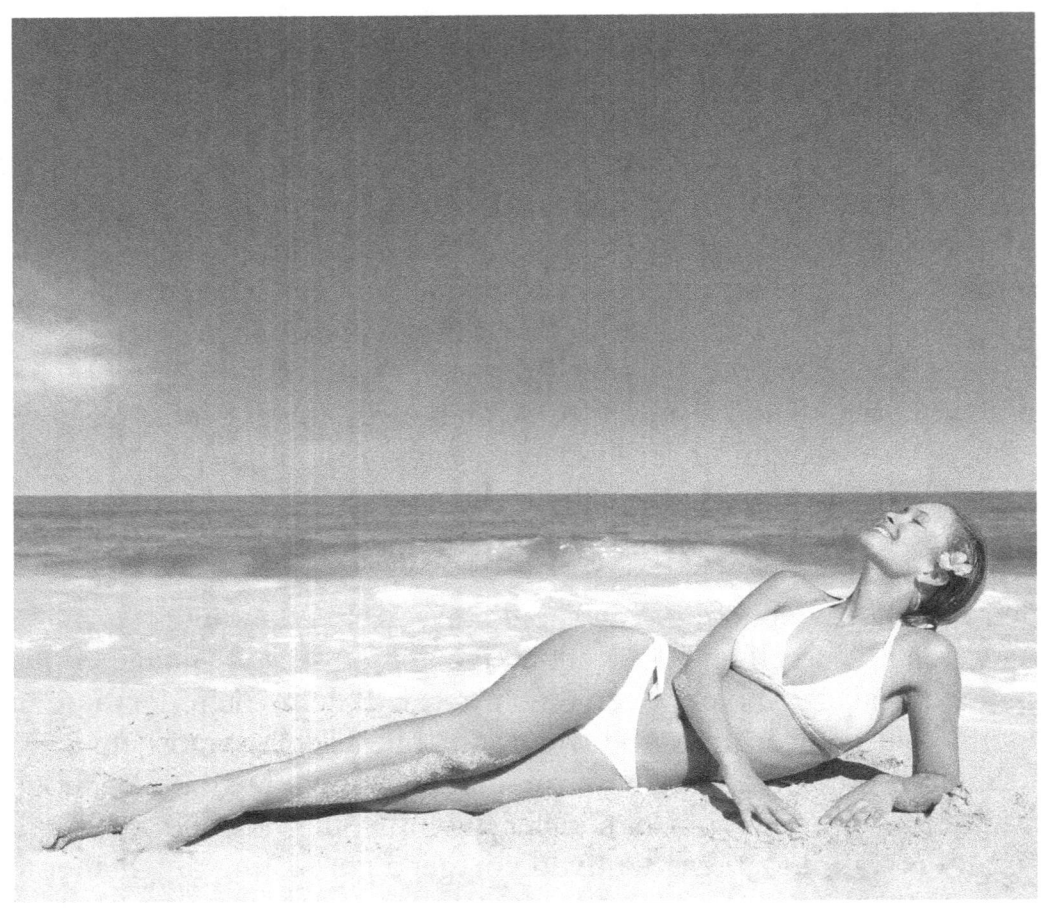

Is tanning your skin a good idea?

Tanning your skin may look healthy and it may make you feel more attractive and sexy, but it is not healthy and it will do you much more harm than good. Just think of what it will do to your skin when you are in the burning hot sun. It changes your color just as it does when you are cooking meat on the barbecue. The older you get, the more wrinkled, dried out and old your skin will look. There is also always the danger of developing skin cancer. You should take time to study your body and keep an eye out for moles and freckles and see what they are doing. Are they changing colors, or is your skin dry or cracked?

Dry skin can be a sign that you need to drink more water or you need to experiment with a different face cream. Taking notice of what your skin is doing is important when keeping in touch with your overall health. Your skin is not just something you have to keep nice and smooth looking, it can also be a sign of what is going on in your body.

What kind of skin care moisturizer do you use?

There is a lot of advice around about using natural products for your cosmetics, and they will tell you to stay away from anything chemical. It doesn't mean that you shouldn't use any product that isn't completely natural, you just need to check what ingredients are in the product you are using. If you get a rash or any kind of skin irritation from it, you should change to another moisturizer which has more natural ingredients and less chemical components in it.

It is not only your moisturizer that you have to be careful of, but some soaps and shampoos have a lot of chemical ingredients in them that can damage sensitive skin. These natural products may cost you a little more, but you will get more value for your money and they will be much kinder to your skin. If you use creams with only natural ingredients in them and you still have skin problems, then you should seek the advice of a dermatologist.

****

How much attention do you pay to any of your senses?

Let us start with the eyes. How much attention do you give your eyes? For many of us it is not something we worry about before we have a problem with them.

The eyes do need to be looked after just like everything else in your body. You have to protect them from too much sun with a good pair of sunglasses that come with UV protection. If you are working in an environment that calls for you wearing goggles, never refuse to wear them because all it takes is a little spark or splash from some chemical stuff to cause major damage to your eyes.

There comes a time when most women can feel their eyesight is not as good as it use to be. There are many things that can cause small changes to your eyesight. Breast feeding can cause temporary changes because of the release of hormones. Your eyes react to stress just like any other part of your body does. When you go through the change of life and you experience hormone changes in your body, it can have an affect on your eyes. Whether you are young or an older woman, you should have your eyes examine on a regular basis. You should not ignore your eyes. Your doctor can prescribe special drops to keep your eyes clear and healthy.

Your throat

Your throat is a very sensitive part of your body. It is from here that you express yourself verbally or hold back what you would really like to say, but don't always have the courage to express. Therefore we might end up with a sore throat and wonder why it is sore. It might be that it is trying to tell you something. There are several reasons for why your throat is sore, and you need to pay attention to it. If it keeps on being sore for days, you should probably go and visit your doctor. Don't hesitate to do that because your doctor will do some tests on your throat and will make sure to give you the right treatment you need to cure your problem.

About Snoring

Snoring has the reputation of being a *male thing*. We imagine a middle aged, overweight man with a tendency to eat or drink too much. It is correct that your diet and intake of too much alcohol and being overweight can cause a person to snore. But it is not only a male thing, anyone can be a snorer. Infants, children and women can have that problem.

Snoring isn't a new problem and people have been looking at ways to silence loud sleeping partners for centuries. Snoring may be common, but it isn't normal. It is indicative of a problem and should be taken seriously. It can take a toll on even the best of relationships; the noise your partner makes when sleeping can cause many sleepless nights for you.

Snoring can be caused by the uvula which is the entity hanging in the back of your throat as well as the soft palate which is the soft spot at the top of your mouth. But these are not the only parts causing you to snore. It can also be your adenoids and tonsils contributing to your snoring. These are just some of the things that cause snoring; there is a selection of different causes such as a narrow throat which often happens as you get older. A restricted airway can be caused if you are carrying too much fat around your neck and therefore encourage snoring.

People who smoke a lot have the potential to snore. The muscles in your throat relax when you smoke and the inhalation of the smoke creates lung and nasal congestion which encourages snoring. This can also be the case with a non smoker living with a smoking partner. Obviously, we have to take snoring seriously. Snoring can be a sign of sleep apnea and the stakes of having that disorder are too high to overlook.

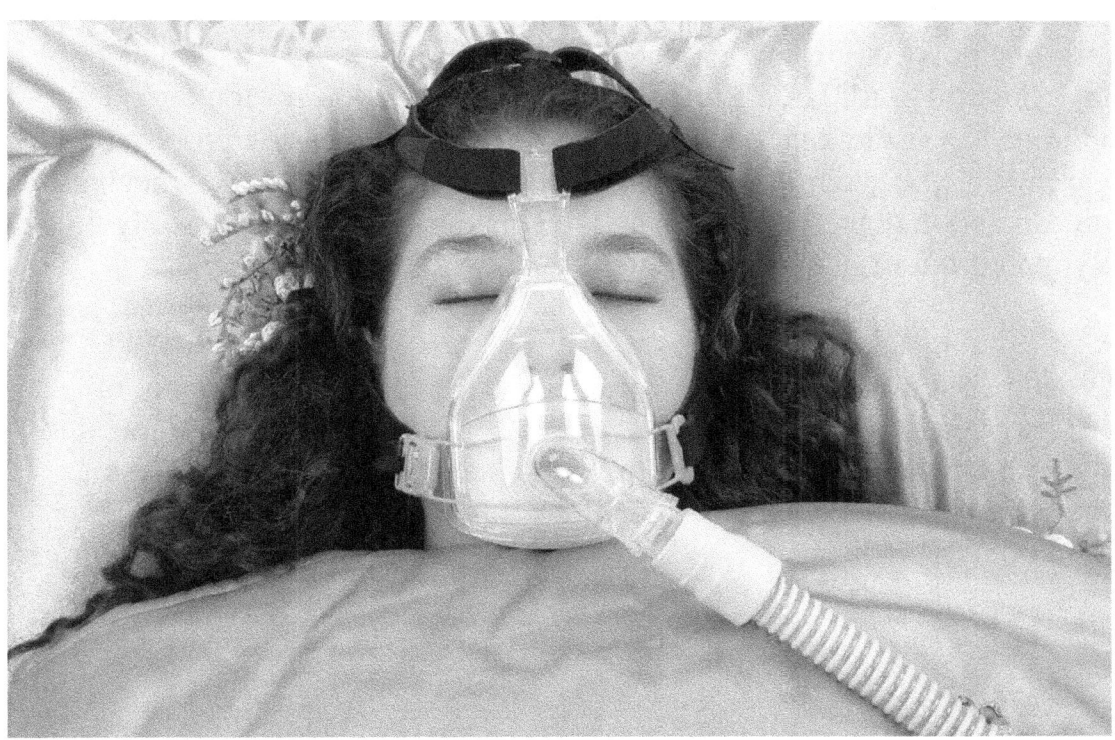

What is sleep apnea?

Sleep apnea refers to breathing difficulty that forces the sufferer to wake up because they have stopped breathing and have to re-start their breathing. The word apnea refers to the absence of breathing, and as frightening as that idea is, it is exactly what happens to many problem snorers. You can actually get a machine from your doctor to help you breath at night. You have it by your bed and it has a mask attach to it which will assist your breathing. This might seem uncomfortable, but when you get used to it, you will appreciate that you get a good undisturbed night's sleep and will wake up more energized than you have for a while, and so will your partner.

There are severe cases when the best way to fix the snoring problem is surgery. This involves removing excess tissues at the back of the throat and taking away any obstacles that cause the snoring, and the uvula itself is also removed. This procedure will result in the widening of the airway and can eliminate snoring altogether for many patients.

Your Ears – keep the volume down

The health of your ears is something you should be looking after. Do you work in a noisy environment where you really should be wearing ear plugs but you don't? Is it because you are afraid it doesn't look good or feminine? Don't let that be the cause of you having hearing problems later in life, you will dearly regret it. Keep the volume down as much as you can and that goes for stereo and television. You should not only think of yourself but of other people around you who will suffer too.

If you are one of those women who goes to the gym and works out or likes to go jogging in the park, but needs to have an earphone strapped to you with a motivating tape to help you to keep up with your exercise, then you should make sure to keep the volume low to protect your ears from too much noise.

****

Breast awareness

We have already talked about how amazing a woman's body is, but it does also have the potential to attract some not so nice malicious illness. So make sure to be attentive in the way you look after your body and do everything you can to stay healthy. Familiarize yourself with how your breasts usually feel so you can be aware of any changes happening with them. The health of your breast is important and you should do a monthly exam. If you find any signs of change in your breasts, you should see your doctor.

Many women are at risk of developing some form of breast cancer over the course of their lives. Early detection is the best and the only way to catch cancer early so that you can still live a reasonably normal life. Therefore, you should carry out a monthly breast exam as part of being a healthy woman as well as your yearly mammograms and gynecological examination.

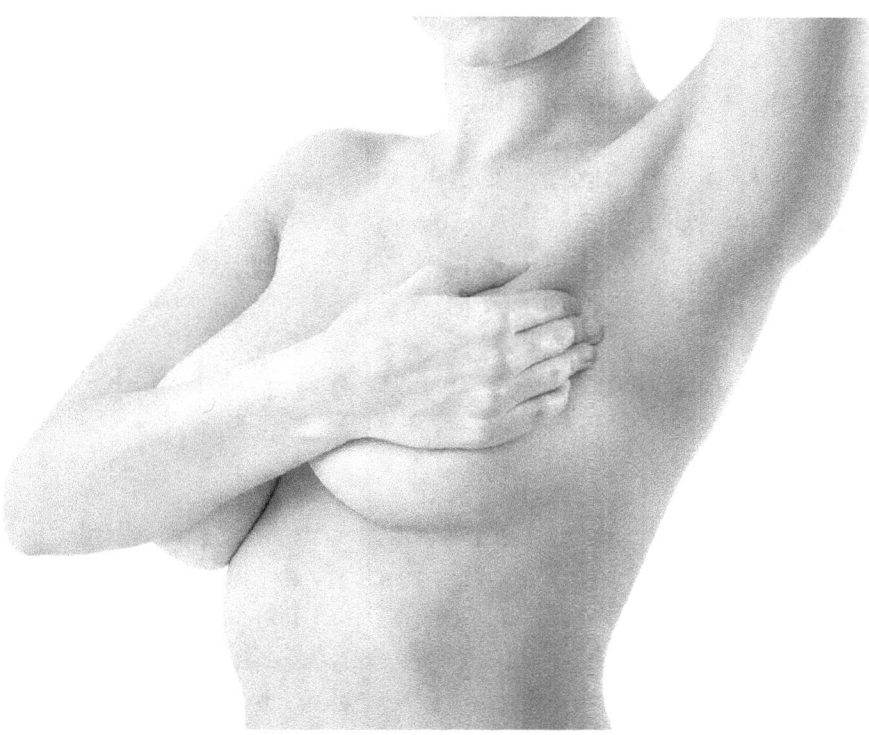

How To - Breast Examination

1. Examine yourself in front of a mirror without your shirt or bra on. Check for any possible changes in the appearance of your skin, shape or texture. This could be in the form of dimpling or puckering.

2. Your nipples should be inspected to ensure that there are no changes in the texture or shape of the skin. You will want to squeeze each one to ensure there is no abnormal discharge.

3. Repeat the first two steps in three additional positions - with your arms at your side, raised over your head and also on your hips.

4. Taking your time, raise one arm and systematically examine the opposite breast (left arm, right breast, etc.) using the pads of your first two fingers. With slight pressure, massage in small circles every inch of your breast feeling for anything abnormal like a bump, lump, thick or fibrous area or even dimpling.

5. Massage under your arm and around the outside of your breast with your fingertips to check for abnormalities.

6. Repeat the systematic examination with the opposite arm and breast.

7. Finally, lay down, placing a pillow under one shoulder, raising that same arm over your head. With the opposite hand, repeat the massage technique to check for lumps and bumps. This gives you a different angle and slightly different search field.

8. Repeat the lie down examination for the opposite side.

When it comes to the breast self-exam, you may use a light lotion to allow your fingers to glide more smoothly around the breast. In addition, choose a particular day of the month in which you do it so that it becomes a long standing habit. Just a note of caution - do not conduct the exam during your period. Instead, wait a few days until after your period when your hormones have had a chance to level out. When you conduct a regular breast examination your chances of an early detection is the key to the successful treatment of breast cancer.

Breastfeeding and health

Breastfeeding is a great way for the baby and mother to bond and it should be encouraged. However there are times when the mother can experience issues while nursing her baby. Breast infections can occur in nursing mothers, and some of them can become quite serious. If you are experiencing anything like that you should seek medical care right away before it gets any worse. An infection such as mastitis can be very painful and needs to be treated with antibiotics.

The medical profession used to state that women who were breastfeeding were protected against breast cancer later in life. However there has been a change of mind about this statement and they no longer believe that is true.

A study has been carried out and they found that breastfeeding can lower your chances for developing breast cancer, but it did not totally rule out the threat. Breastfeeding is a wonderful way of providing food for your baby but just keep in mind that problems can come up and it is important that you stay healthy.

****

Your heart - how healthy is your heart

If you suffer from heart problems then it is something you should be concerned about, take serious and seek the advice of your doctor. Heart disease can be a real danger to women and if your doctor advises you to exercise, eat right or go on a special diet, you should really listen to what your doctor tells you to do.

Your doctor is only trying to help you to stay as healthy as possible and reduce your risks of heart failure. If you are on any special prescription medication and you are having heart problems, then you need to make sure that it is safe to take with your heart condition. You need to be alert as to what medication your doctor prescribes for you. Doctors often consult a lot of patients and therefore you need to refresh his memories about your medical condition. Don't ever take for granted that your doctor remembers all the conditions you may have, so make sure to keep your ears and eyes open to what goes on with your health.

Both men and women can be subject to having a heart attack and it can be due to many different situations such as stress or being overweight. But in these cases it should be remembered that perhaps it could have been avoided if the person had taken the time to looked a bit deeper into the psychological side of things and found out why they suffered from stress and why they were overweight? What personal issues do these people have that caused them to have heart problems?

Divorce and a broken relationship that leaves you with a broken heart can have a severe effect on a person both physically and emotionally. The loss of a loved one can be hard to cope with and the person left behind needs to allow time to grieve.

If any traumatic experience is not dealt with emotionally and suppressed, the person's feelings will most probably show up in other ways through the body. Emotional experiences need time to heal and should be treated with loving tender care.

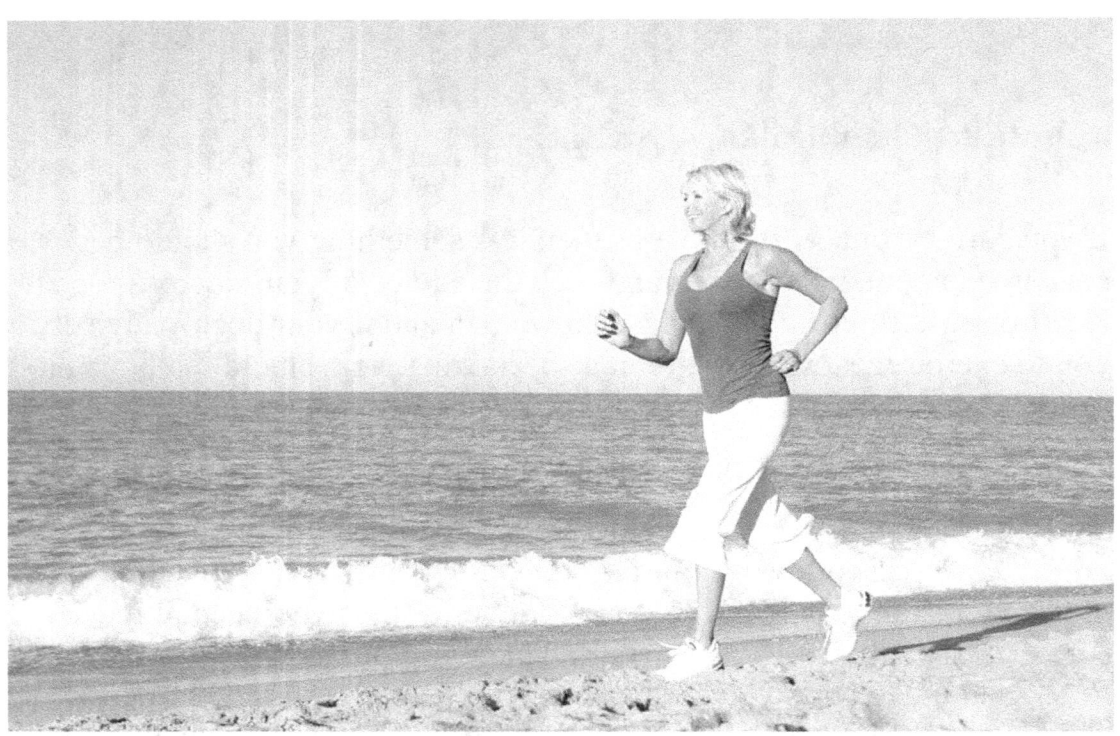

Exercise is important for your health

When you exercise your body you are giving your heart a workout too. Think about how well you will feel after having exercised regularly for a while and the benefit your heart gets too. When your body works efficiently, the easier it is for the heart to pump the blood through the body. Even if heart disease doesn't run in the family, you still have to exercise to keep your heart healthy.

If you are a person who is not very active or sits down a lot, then your heart has to work a lot harder to get the blood to pump through your body. Even if you are not into heavy workouts or keeping fit, you owe it to yourself to exercise for the benefit of your heart. You don't have to be too hard on yourself but start off with a simple walk around the block early in the morning or after your dinner and then slowly increase your walk a little longer, but no more than you feel comfortable with.

A woman's bladder is a sensitive area

To avoid a bladder infection, make sure you drink plenty of water or any kind of fluid. It is also suggested that cranberry juice can be a healing substance to take. A bladder infection can be very painful and if you experience a burning feeling when you urinate then you should seek treatment from your doctor. If you are not sure about what is wrong but you are having a feeling of wanting to urinate and you only get small dribbles coming out, you should get a sample of your urine tested by your doctor who will send it to the lab for further examination. If the test confirms that you have a bladder infection, your doctor will prescribe some antibiotics that will treat the infection. If you have any other problems in these areas, it is best to talk to your doctor and follow his advice on how to treat these ailments.

****

Most women know how to eat healthy – so why don't we?

We have all heard that an *apple a day keeps the doctor away*. We also know that we have to eat healthy and make sure we get plenty of fruits and vegetables in our diet. Maybe you are one of those people who does stick to eating healthy, but there are many people who don't. What is the reason for people not sticking to a healthy diet when we know that it is best for our bodies and it will function much better if we follow a healthy diet?

Are you addicted to certain sweets or do you have a habit of eating fast food, maybe because it is easier than cooking a meal for yourself? That is a bad habit. You should always try to eat as healthy as possible. Your body needs healthy food and there is no magic age when it's an ideal time to get healthy, although the earlier you begin the more likely it will become a habit throughout your lifetime and much more beneficial to you overall. There is also no age that you can reach where there is simply no point in trying to be healthy, because this is a noble aspiration at any age.

Women's health is different from men's health, but one thing does unify both men and women: the more effort you put into being healthy, the more your body will reward you with strength, stamina, and longevity. It's important to remember that you are solely responsible for your health. Find a way that is important enough for you to change your eating habit in order to eat healthy.

Your kidney and medication

There is something you need to know about medication that you may not ever have thought about. Every medicine and drug you ingest has to go through your kidneys! Taking too much medication can actually damage your kidneys. Most women are on some sort of medical prescription from their doctor at one time or another. You may also be on some sort of over the counter drugs that you take occasionally or perhaps you take some vitamin pills as well. All these pills that you are hoping will keep you healthy may in fact react to each other in some way and do you more harm than good. Everything in moderation, if it is possible you should cut back on the amount of pills you take at the same time.

****

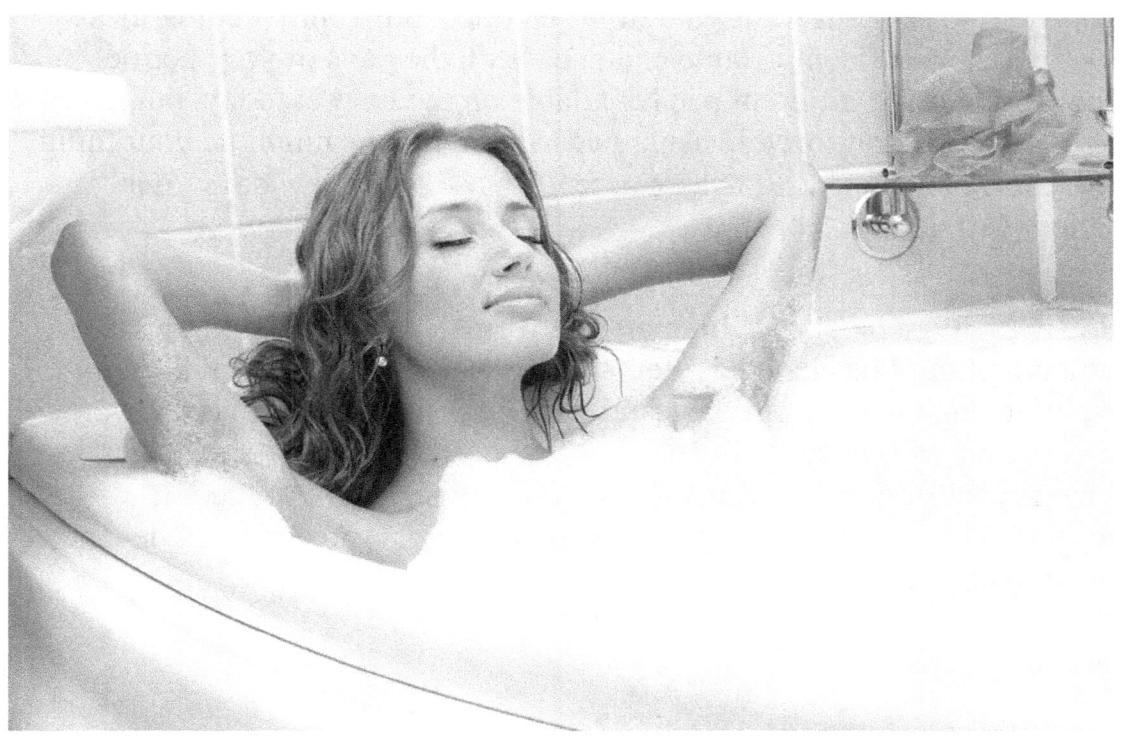

Are you in touch with your femininity?

Sometimes our everyday life calls for us women to do things that are not necessarily very feminine but it is expected of us simply just to get by in our lives. But then there comes a time when it feels great to be a woman; we can dress up in a pretty dress and smart shoes and look really feminine which makes you feel like a woman. Women need to care for themselves now and again, like relax in a hot bath for a long time and then cover yourself in a good body lotion. Caring for yourself in that way gets you in touch with not only the feminine part of you, but also the goddess within you, and that is so important because that will also awaken the creativity in you.

Certain part of a woman's body require more attention

It must be remembered that even though all women are different in some ways then we must bear in mind that we all have to tend to the female parts of our bodies, such as breast self-exams and our menstrual cycles. It is wise to see a medical professional now and again if only to be encouraged to pay attention to our female parts. It can be pretty annoying for a woman to have to put up with her monthly period.

You want to find out what kind of protection from your bleeding makes you feel the most comfortable and at ease on the days of your period. There are a lot of different pads available on the market today, but if you are not feeling comfortable using pads then tampons might be your thing. The choice is yours as long as you feel at ease in the few days your periods lasts.

However, hygiene plays a big part in a woman's health and your pad or tampons should be changed often and not worn all day. If you keep on experiencing bleeding for days and days, you should pay a visit to your doctor who will most likely take some test. There are things that can be done if your periods are causing you to feel sick and not function normally, but the treatment your doctor will suggest to you will depend on what age you are at.

Watch which area of your body you spray perfume

A woman's vagina is a delicate area of the body and many women worry about bad odor, therefore spraying themselves with perfume or some scented spray around this area. It is not a good idea to use chemical products in this area, think of the damage it can have on the inside of your body. If you do have a bad odor coming from your vagina, it is time to visit your doctor. You could have some sort of infection which can easily be treated with medication.

****

Fashion and Health

How many of us women have suffered just to follow the fashion of today. That has happened for centuries, women would go to extremes just to be looking trendy and wearing what was considered fashionable even if they had to suffer wearing clothes that were too tight. Are we getting any wiser? I still see young women walking around in huge high heel shoes looking very uncomfortable and never giving a thought to what it is doing to their health.

I understand it makes a young woman feel attractive to wear the latest fashion even if it means putting on a tight pair of jeans so tight that she can hardly breathe and frilly uncomfortable underwear.

Most women like to dress up once in a while and make themselves look beautiful, which is really good for your self-esteem. It is sort of an assurance that you are a good looking woman. However, you should take into consideration that some of the fashionable clothing is not very good for your health. Wearing a pair of too tight jeans and frilly underwear that makes you feel uncomfortable, for any length of time can cause you to develop an infection in your vagina. Your vagina needs air now and again but if you dress in too tight underwear then your vagina gets deprived from the air it needs and you could end up with yeast infection.

What many women don't realize is that when they are wearing high heeled shoes, their body is actually getting out of balance and it can cause back problems. Women are expected to look fabulous in whatever job they do even if it is not healthy for them. You will see when there is some big fancy celebration of the stars (who are usually the trend setters) wearing all those beautiful low cut and expensive dresses and they must be freezing cold sometimes while the men are dressed in a nice and warm suit!

We have probably all been guilty of not dressing sensibly because we wanted to wear a special gorgeous thin dress to some event that was important to us and frozen our butts off, and worn fabulous but uncomfortable high heels shoes. We should really stop and take a look at how we dress and ask ourselves is it healthy the way we dress?

We need to protect our bodies against the elements

Women all over the world have to cope with all kinds of weather and in some places it can be extremely cold or hot. The different elements can be pretty harmful to your body and therefore you need to protect it against the hot sun, wind and the freezing cold winters. When you are exposed to too much sun, your skin will become dry and you will end up looking old before your time if you don't wear sun screen lotion and protective clothing.

When you know that you will be exposed to the sun for any length of time you should wear a hat, a long sleeved top and long pants. It is wise to dress according to what the weather is like. In the colder climate it makes sense to dress in clothes that protect you against the cold weather. If you live in a climate where the temperature gets way below zero and the frost sets in, you should make sure to cover your face with a good moisturizer to protect it against frostbite.

Maintain good health

You may have good health now but you do need to look after your health if you want it to last. There are many beverages and foods that you may be better off avoiding. Consume everything in moderation if you want to keep on enjoying good health. Drinking a lot of coffee or any caffeinated drinks during the day can be bad for you. It may boost your ability to think quicker and more clearly, however it only last for a while and you may become more and more dependent on your caffeine drink throughout the day to give you a boost to keep going.

There is nothing wrong with a few cups of coffee during your day but it is when you start to rely on coffee so it becomes an addiction, your body will suffer. If you are relying on any sort of caffeinated drinks and you decide to give it up completely then you will most probably experience withdrawing symptoms such as headaches and moodiness. If you cut back on your caffeine slowly then it will not be as bad, but that is an individual choice. Whichever way you decide to give it up, the end result will definitely be worth it because you will feel free from your addiction.

The same goes for alcohol. Drinking too much alcohol can easily become an addiction. A sociable drink of alcohol is alright but it is when you make it a daily habit and need a drink of alcohol to get you through the day that it becomes a concern. Most alcohol has a high amount of calories, so it could also add more weight to your body. The influence of alcohol can be a tricky thing for some people who have a history of alcoholism in their family. According to some doctors, alcoholism can be heredity. What starts out as a sociable drink for them now and again can develop into a serious drinking problem. You need to take a look at your individual situation and decide if indulging in alcohol is in your best interest when it comes to your health.

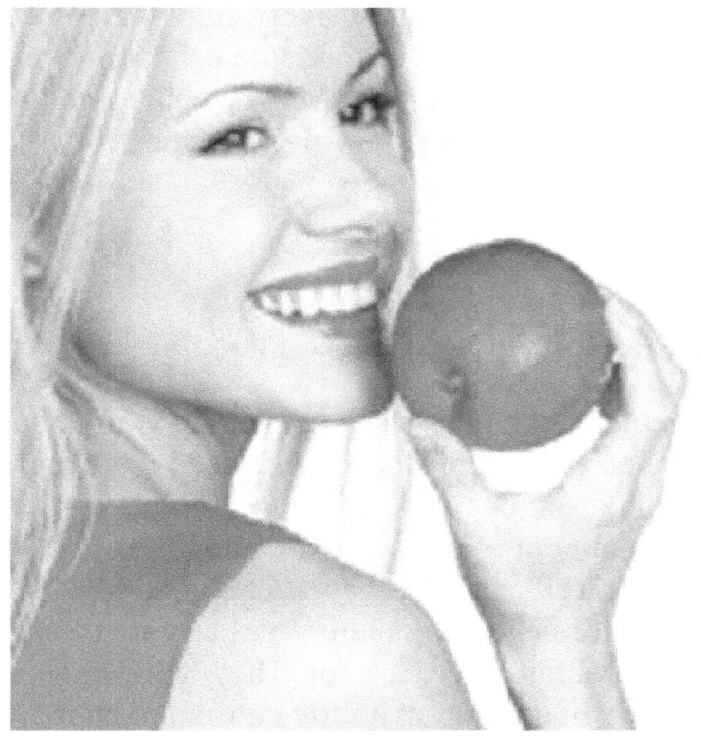

Nutrients in your food are important for your health

Get into the habit of eating healthy food and do some form of exercise often. The sooner you start, the better it is for you. It doesn't matter what age you are when you start, but the younger you are the more you will benefit when you get older. To maintain a healthy body, you require certain nutrients and vitamins. It is very fashionable to be thin but you want to be careful with some diet that excludes good wholesome foods from your menu or you may end up ill.

If you decide to go on a diet, you should consult a professional dietitian to be on the safe side. Being skinny does not necessarily mean being healthy. Women comes in all shapes and sizes and some bodies are not meant to be really skinny and will make the person unhealthy and even ill if losing too much weight. You need to learn to become aware of how your body is functioning. If you are on a diet and you feel your energy level is dropping, then you are probably not getting the nutrients your body needs.

It is crucial to keep yourself in balance in body, mind and spirit. If you need to loose a lot of weight, then you should do so with a professional medical practitioner's help who will give you a sensible and healthy diet plan to follow. But if you are not hugely overweight then you should just attempt to cut down on the portions of food you eat and make sure that you are physically active during the day. Make a habit of taking a good walk every day or even visit a gym a few times a week for a good workout.

To maintain good health you need to get a good night's sleep

It is important to get a good night's sleep to keep up your good health. We don't all need the same amount of sleep. Some need more and others need less. Each individual person has to be the judge of what is right for them. However it is important not to skip whatever amount of sleep your body and mind needs to feel well and refreshed after a good night's sleep. Women are notorious for neglecting themselves and are often deprived from sleep if they have a family to care for. They will always make sure that everyone is tucked in bed and that little household chores are done before they go to bed. If you are a young mother and have just had a baby and breast feeding, then you are going to have to get up during the night to feed the baby in the beginning. There is a lot to get used to until you get the baby into a routine and you will probably be sleep deprived unless you have someone to help you out with the chores while you catch up on some sleep.

What ever your reason is for lack of sleep; partying, working hard, studying too late at night, your risk of getting sick and catching cold are much higher than normal. Your reaction to your surroundings is slowed down, you become irritable and don't function as well as you would when you have had a good night's sleep. Your body needs sleep. It is healing for your soul and body. Many times when we have a problem that we are trying to solve but can't find an answer to it, then a good night sleep will help and you often wake up with a clear mind and you now know what to do about your problem.

Women have different needs according to their age

Most women's bodies function well when they are young but as they get older their bodies can't cope with the same treatment we gave it when we were young. Not too many young women think about their body as something they should look after and often don't give a second thought. Their body is not going to be in good condition forever if they don't treat it well.

If you don't take care of your body now while you are young and watch how much alcohol, smokes, and fast food you consume, you can be in real trouble as you get older. Any damage you inflict on your body at a young age can have a lasting affect on your health. Your youth should be enjoyed but you have to know your limits not to overindulge to the detriment of your health. By getting into the habit of eating healthy and living a healthy lifestyle while you are young, will be one of the best investments you can do for yourself, it will pay off when you get older.

When is a good time to start a family?

Many women chose to start a family a lot later in life these days. They want to enjoy their youth, get a good education so they can have a career of their choice and get the feel of being independent. A lot of women are not ready to have a family before they are in their thirties. If you are one of these women then you should make sure that your health is the best it can be before you get pregnant. That way your pregnancy will be a lot easier to cope with.

If you are a bit overweight then try to get to the weight that you are most comfortable with. Find time to exercise and take multi-vitamins with folic acid before you get pregnant. A baby can be a lot of work especially if it is your first born. You need to stay healthy and keep your energy up in order to care for your baby. So if you are smoking and drinking then stop, it is bad for the baby's health as well as your own.

****

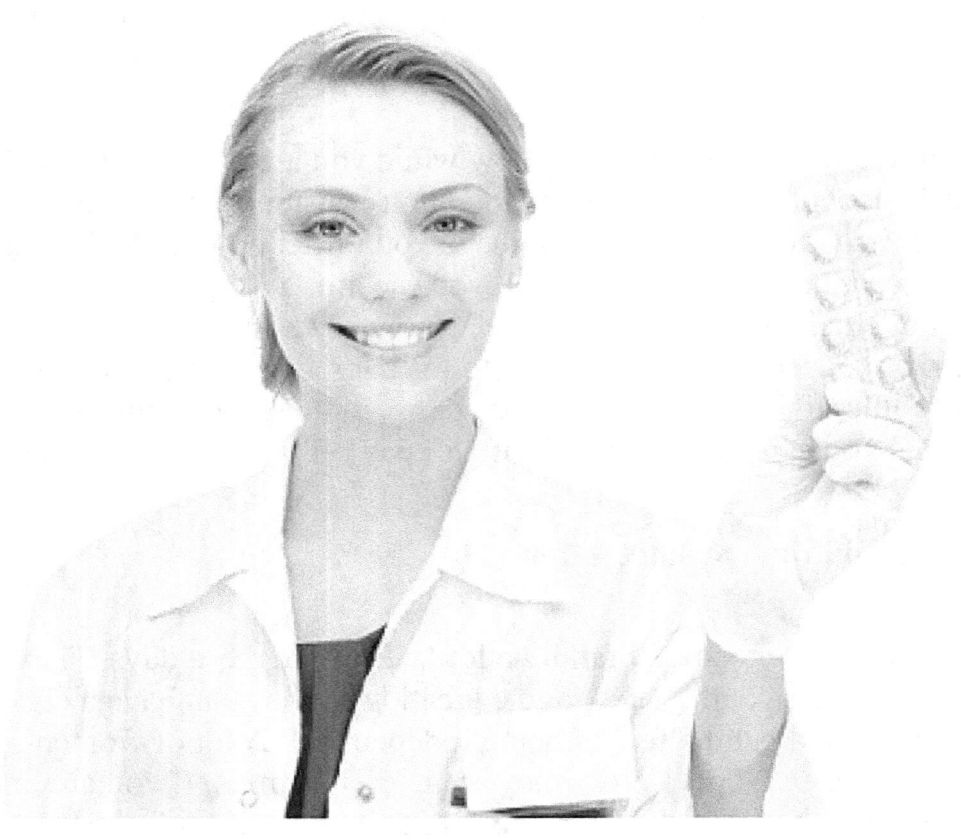

Birth control pills

Have you enjoyed having safe sex while being on birth control pills for a long time? Then what you may not realize is that there may come a time when your body starts to react to these pills and your emotions start to get a little out of control. You should talk to your doctor about how you now react to the birth control pill and he can help you to find some alternate forms of pills or perhaps a lower dose to get your body and emotions into balance again. If you are going through emotional ups and downs, make sure that it isn't the birth control pill that is causing you to be out of balance.

Be prepare for the change of life

Even though you are still a beautiful woman your body may begin to show small sign of aging. You may start to get a few small wrinkles and a few grey hairs. This may worry some women but try to adopt a positive mind set and look at yourself as a healthy woman in the prime of your life. It is inevitable not to age. It happens to all of us, but when you embrace the unavoidable with an optimistic attitude, when the signs of peri-menopause start to take affect you will be able to handle it much better. If you have a healthy frame of mind it will also have a positive affect on your physical body.

Peri-menopause

Peri-menopause is when the body start to prepare for menopause and the change of life. The signs may be subtle and in many cases women may not even be aware of the changes happening and will put them down to other things causing the affects it has on you. Some women may start to show early signs of peri-menopause; their periods become irregular and they could suffer other strange symptoms.

The early 50's are the average age for women to experience Menopause so you could be starting with the symptoms of Menopause during your 40's and for some women even sooner. Changes in your menstrual cycle are the most common indication that is leading up to Menopause but it could also be misinterpreted. There are some signs of the beginning of Menopause that you could recognize but there could also be other factors involved. Some of the symptoms are the following. Fibroids, cysts, cancer, and a host of other factors can also cause changes, so get a gynecological exam to make sure you are in good health.

Body temperature fluctuations such as night sweats are common as well as hot flashes that typical last just a few seconds. As you creep closer to full-blown menopause, these episodes will last longer. Some women actually get cold sweats and are more prone to outer temperature changes during menopause. Mood swings are often an indicator that menopause has started to take effect. Being overly sensitive, anxious, irritable or even depressed are early signs of menopause that many women report feeling. Vaginal issues are some of the symptoms that women can experience before menopause. Their natural vaginal lubrication is greatly decreased due to the lower estrogen production prior to menopause. Lubrication products may have to be purchased if dryness is a major problem.

Along with sleep issues peri-menopause causes hormone fluctuations, which can contribute to problems of trying to fall asleep or even staying asleep. The night sweats are part of the sleep problem as well. Memory and concentration may not be as good as they use to be. Where once you could remember most details, you now have to write everything down. Feeling scattered is another issue prior to menopause and concentration can be difficult. These issues are caused by hormonal changes in the body. You can overcome this by increasing your vitamin B intake to maintain better health and more able to cope with the situation. Basically, peri-menopause has symptoms that are quite similar to menopause, only to a lesser degree.

The true sign of the switch from peri-menopause to the real deal is the lack of a period for over a year, barring any other health issues. While not every woman experiences symptoms during the lead up to menopause for other women symptoms can wreak havoc for ten years or even longer.

Early menopause

Early menopause is a term often used in the time leading up to the full blown menopause. If you experience early menopause symptoms at an earlier than normal age, but are still ovulating and have your hormone levels tested at normal levels, you'll sometimes be told you're in early menopause. This is a period of time leading up to menopause and it can take as long as 10 to 15 years. Your menstrual cycle becomes unpredictable and you could suffer from odd symptoms. This can come well before the average age of normal menopause. For some women it can come when you are still in your 20s, 30s, or early 40s. Early menopause can be emotionally devastating and can become a health problem for some women.

When does menopause start?

Menopause begins when a woman stops ovulating and her monthly menstruation stops. Most women reach menopause between the ages of 45 and 55. There are about one per cent of women who experience menopause before the age of 40 years. This is known as early menopause or premature ovarian failure. The symptoms of early menopause are the same as menopause and can include menstrual cycle changes, hot flushes, sweats, urinary problems such as incontinence or increased frequency of urination, dry vagina, mood changes and weight changes. Early menopause means the woman's ovaries have spontaneously stopped working before she has reached the age of 40 years. There is no treatment available to make the ovaries start working again. Women with early menopause have a long period of post-menopausal life, and there is the risk of health problems such as osteoporosis and heart disease. It may be a good idea to join a support group with women who are also experiencing early menopause. For some women it can happen that their ovaries suddenly start to work again and according to some studies, about one in 10 women who are diagnosed with unnatural early menopause get pregnant, for reasons that are not yet clear.

What is menopause?

What exactly is menopause itself? It simply means that menopause is the stop of your periods. Your periods stop because your ovaries have run out of eggs and are no longer responding to your body's hormonal signals. They may have been damaged or been surgically removed. Before your periods stops, you go through a transition period called peri-menopause.

This can last on average from two to six years, although some women have it for a shorter amount of time, and others longer. And once your periods have stopped for a year, you're considered as being in menopause.

Many middle age women don't start to think about their health before they get into the menopause cycle. If they had started the habit of healthy living earlier then they would have coped better with their change of life. Of course many women have looked well after themselves and are now reaping the benefit.

With age comes wisdom

As you get older you become wiser, and many women get a lot better idea of who they are as a person and what they want out of life. They don't worry so much about what other people think of them or if they get a few grey hairs or a few extra pounds along the way. Even though you are not a youngster anymore it can still be a good feeling to be a mature woman.

However with the beginning of menopause you might experience some uncomfortable symptoms and some women decide to follow the doctor's advice and settle for estrogens replacement therapy to help them through these unpleasant symptoms.

You should talk to your doctor and make sure it is going to be the right thing for you to take. There has been research done that proved a certain risks involved when taken estrogens replacement therapy that it could increase the chances for some serious illnesses. You should ask plenty of questions and do your own researches before you decide whether to go on estrogens replacement therapy or not.

Get Healthy

It should be remembered that even though age is creeping up on you, it is never too late to get healthy. Watching what you eat and exercising is a good way to start but just like with younger women, you need to take care when you start on new exercises. You have to start slowly and realize that you are much more prone to injuries when you are older and you take a lot longer to heal. That doesn't mean that you are too old to start something new in the form of exercises, you just have to be careful. You may also find as you get older that your choice of food may change and it could be your body telling you or leading you on the path to healthier eating.

Many women get bored eating the same food all the time so it is important that you keep on adding variety to your food rather than eating the same kinds of food over and over again. Not changing the selection of the food you eat may lead you off the path of eating healthy and that is a mistake you do not want to make. Buy some cook books, borrow some from your local library or look for good healthy recipes on the Internet. There are plenty of options to choose from. The other part of being healthy is doing exercise which is very important even if you just go for a walk every day around the block for a start. Later on when you are getting into the habit of walking you can extend your walk a little at the time.

How do you keep on being motivated to do the exercises? Just like your eating healthy needs to be made more exciting, you also need to keep the excitement alive when it comes to your exercise. If you get bored walking alone you could invite a friend along or you could join a the local fitness center where you can interact with other motivated mature women who will help keep the excitement alive, which is important for your overall health. It does take some work on your part, but a combination of eating healthy and exercise is sure to spell success.

Being healthy as you get older can also mean the difference in being independent and dependent. It is good to know that you have supportive family and friends around you but you do not want to have to rely on them for their support all the time. So making sure you stay as healthy as possible is important and there is no reason why you should not be able to do that if you can possibly avoid diseases, illness and injuries. Don't feel that because you are now what we could call a senior citizen that it is too late for you to improve your health, it is always a good time to improve your health.

Many women live until they are in their late eighties or nineties these days. This means that if you are seventy now, you could have another twenty years left to live and you want them to be happy healthy years. They can be if you make a point of taken care of your health and become as healthy as you possibly can be. Age is no excuse to stop taking care of your health and it doesn't have to be hard you just have to follow some general guide lines.

Make sure to be active, do exercises and eat healthy.

You know smoking is no good for you so stop smoking.

Only drink alcohol in moderation.

Don't take drugs; only what your doctor prescribes for you.

Make sure and eat plenty of fruits and vegetables.

Stay away from too much fatty food.

Make sure to get a good night's sleep every night.

Learn to relax and keep your stress level down.

Unprotected sex can get you in trouble, so avoid it.

Following the list above will help to make you healthier at whatever age you are at. It is just a matter of changing your old habits and taking on some healthier habits. Take action; be responsible for your own health. You are the one that has to be in control of the kind of lifestyle you lead and the one who makes the decision to stay healthy. It is good to have someone to support you but you really have to want to be in good health yourself or it is not going to work for you.

Have you inherited a disease that runs in the family?

If some of your family members have a certain disease and it may be something that runs in the family, it can be in the genes of some of the family members, but that does not mean that you have it. However you should look into your family's medical history and see what you can learn from it. It might help you to want to keep healthy as there are some diseases you can avoid simply by living healthy.

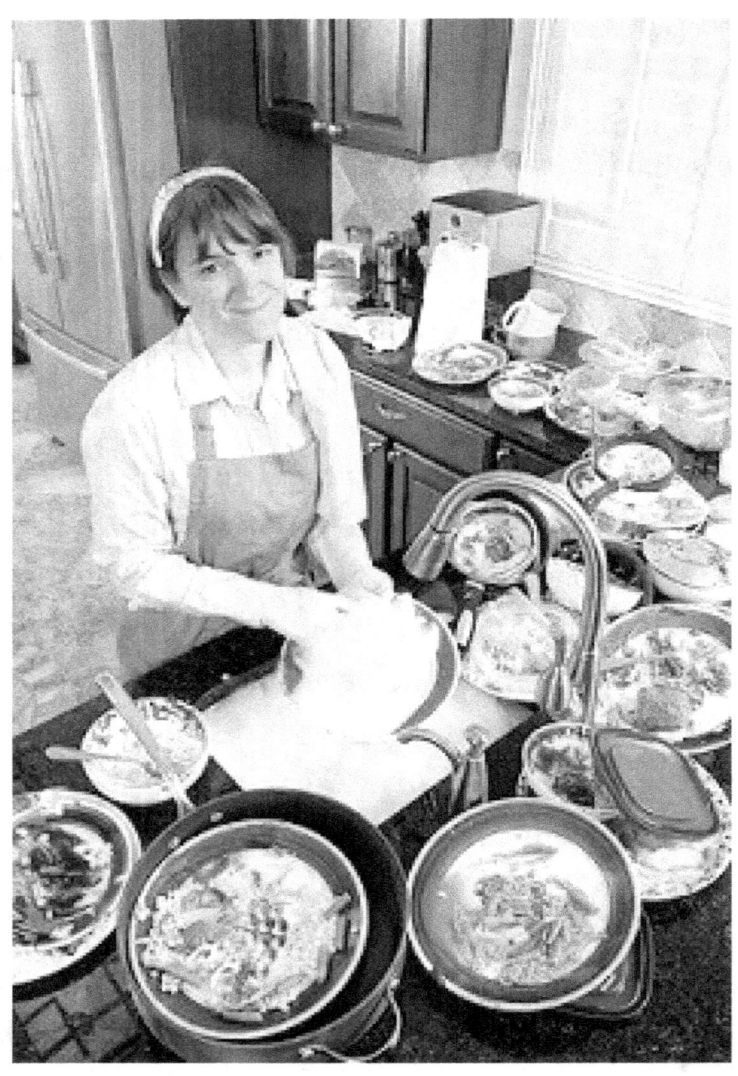

The average woman usually has a big workload

Why are women trying to prove that they can handle it all? We take on every chore in the household and often get the job done really fast. Is it in our genes or is it because we are able to do more than one thing at the same time, whereas men can only handle one thing at the time? We will be doing the washing and the dishes in between while we often have a baby or a small toddler on one arm at the same time as we are cooking a meal.

Women need to have some time off for themselves now and again if they don't want to run themselves down and do damage to their health. Stress is more often than not directly connected to your health and when we are stressed about something we are more prone to pick up any illness going around.

Too much stress will eventually get to you one way or the other and people can see the physical affect it has on you. You may get dark shadows under your eyes and your face will look unhealthy and break out in a rash. Some women might gain weight as a result of being stressed out. Being stressed on a regular basis due to either worries or work overload can have a physiological effect on your body, stress is definitely bad for your health.

Keeping yourself active and busy is not a bad thing. It is when it takes over your life and you don't take time out to relax now and again that it can be a danger to your health. If this is an issue in your life, you need to recognize the harm it can cause you. How can you expect to be healthy if you keep pushing yourself beyond your limits?

Are you so used to being busy that you simply can't stop your busy lifestyle and you wouldn't know how to relax or what to do with yourself if you weren't active all the time? So why should you slow down now? There are many explanations why you should slow down and your health and mental stability are some of the reasons. Slowing down and working at a slower pace would certainly benefit your health. Being healthy is not only about eating healthy and exercise; it is also about how much stress you allow into your life and how you are able to deal with it.

Do you have a family who constantly needs your attention?

If you are a mother and have a few kids, your stress level will be high at times. There will be nights where you don't get much sleep because one of the kids is sick or crying because of teething problems. Most moms do their best but it sure takes a toll on their health if they jump around trying to meet everyone's needs in the family. It might be time to teach the older kids to be more independent and do little chores around the house for you, which they might even enjoy. It will be better for your health to share some of your work load with your family and they will be better off with a mom and a wife who is healthy rather than a worn out woman.

Whether you are a young woman, middle aged or an older woman, it is important to take responsibility for your own health. There are a lot of responsibilities that fall on a woman's shoulders and it can be exhausting at times. So if you don't take responsibilities for yourself and take time out to look after yourself now and again then you might find that a lot of work will simply be dumped on you. You have to learn to say NO and let others do their share of the work.

It is usually the woman who becomes the caretaker of someone in need. You might have an elderly parent who needs your help or kids or grandkids that need your constant attention. You might be a person who takes it all onboard because you think it is your duty as a woman to care for everyone. You need to stop and think about yourself because chances are that you are probably feeling worn out and stressed out if you allow yourself to take on too many responsibilities. If you are in that situation as a woman, it is time to find a balance between your work and finding time to take care of yourself; which means having some free time where you do what you want for yourself. Whether it is having time out with your girlfriends or simply enjoying some relaxation time for yourself without feeling guilty, tell yourself that you too deserve to be cared for.

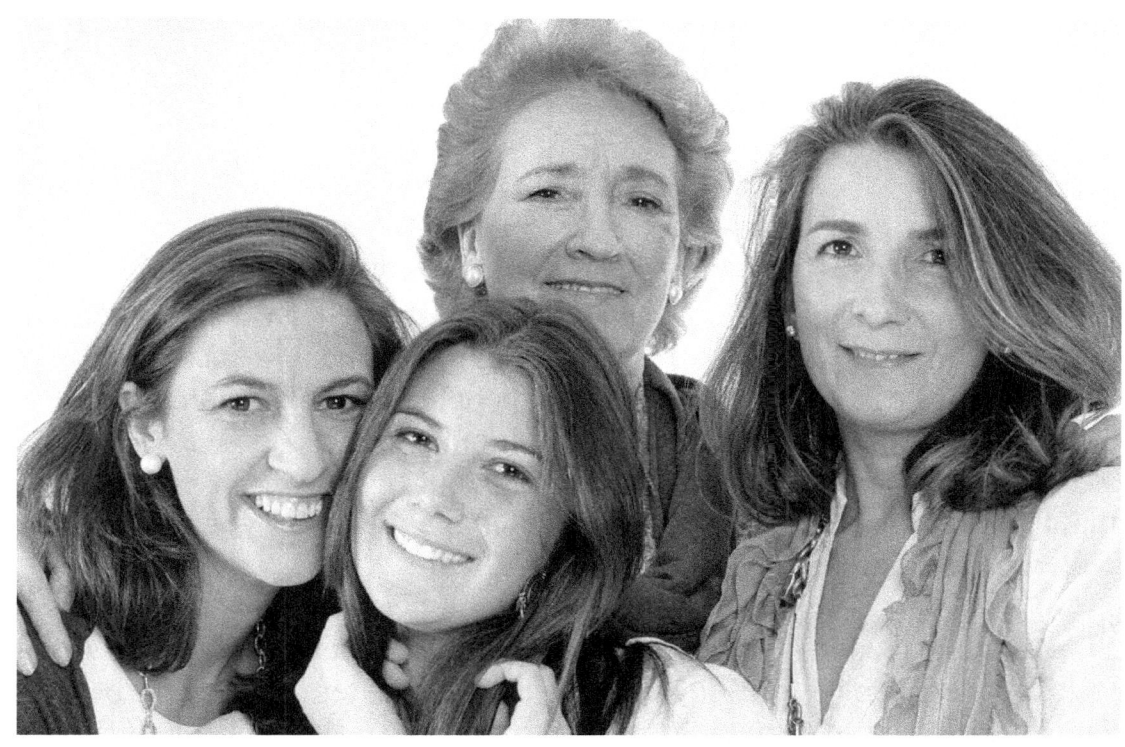

Girlfriends

Most women need a few good girlfriends or at least one close girlfriend
that they can confide in and share personal and private things with.
Families are great but you should always have girlfriends that you can
share a good laugh with and do girly fun things together. It can help lift
your spirit when you are feeling a bit down to share your problems over a
latte with your friend and she might even tell you that she has been
through the same situation and worked through it and now she feels so
much stronger because of it. So cherish your girlfriends and stay in
contact with them where ever your life's journey may take you, and you
can be friends for the rest of your life.

The final word

We are all responsible for our own health and the better we look after our bodies the more it will pay off by giving you good health, energy and strength. You can seek out professional people to help you and it might motivate you for a while, but in the end it really comes down to how willing you are to take responsibilities for your own health. Keep in mind that the more recharged and energized you are, the better you will cope with whatever situation you are presented with.

Stop making excuses and begin to care about your health. The sooner you start to take responsibilities for your health, the better off you will be. Think of it as an investment in yourself that will reward you handsomely. Set a goal for yourself and stick to it. What would you like life to be like one year from now? Do you want to loose a certain amount of weight or do you just want to feel better and healthier? Whatever it is you want for yourself, you can achieve it if you put your mind to it.

This Book is

Published by Dane Print publication

and

Written

By

Tara Collins

If you enjoy reading this Book you may want to tell your friends about it and share the information from the Book with them, and please leave a review. Below is the link to Dane Print Books where you will also find other published books

http://daneprintbooks.com/blog/tips-for-women-to-stay-healthy/